THE PICT
HYMNS

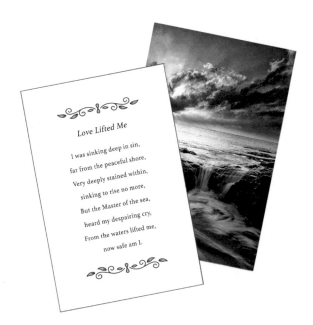

Love Lifted Me

I was sinking deep in sin,
far from the peaceful shore,
Very deeply stained within,
sinking to rise no more,
But the Master of the sea,
heard my despairing cry,
From the waters lifted me,
now safe am I.

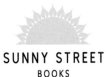

SUNNY STREET
BOOKS

Shall We Gather at the River?

Shall we gather at the river,

Where bright angel feet have trod,

With its crystal tide forever

Flowing by the throne of God?

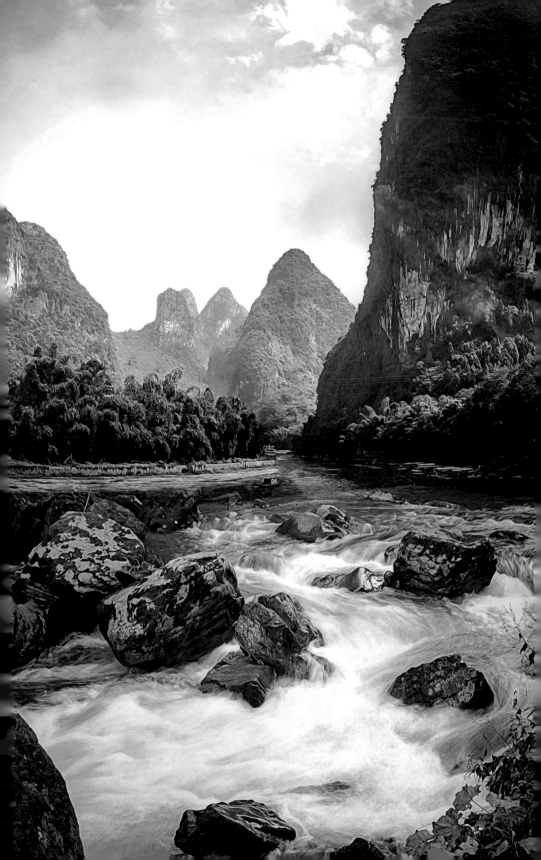

In the Garden

And he walks with me,

And he talks with me,

And he tells me I am His own;

And the joy we share

as we tarry there,

None other has ever known.

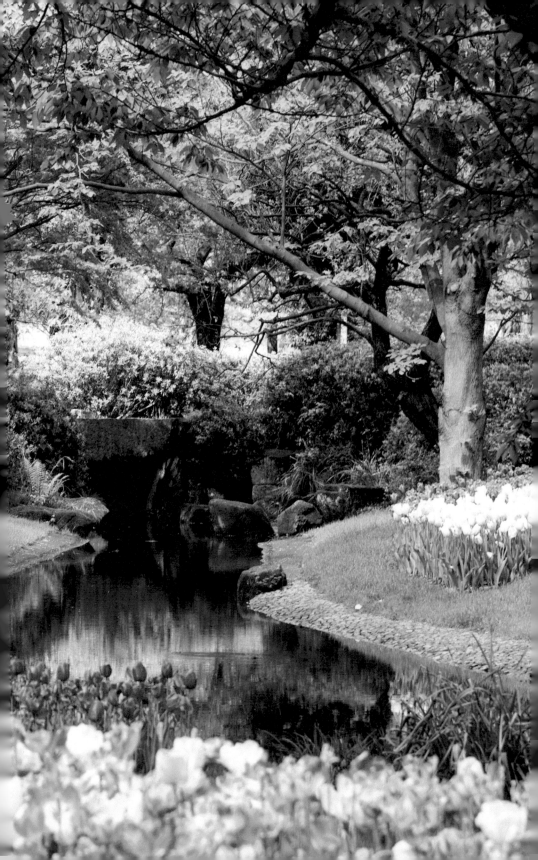

Rock of Ages

Rock of Ages, cleft for me,

Let me hide myself in Thee.

Let the water and the blood,

From Thy wounded side which flowed.

Be of sin the double cure;

Save from wrath and make me pure.

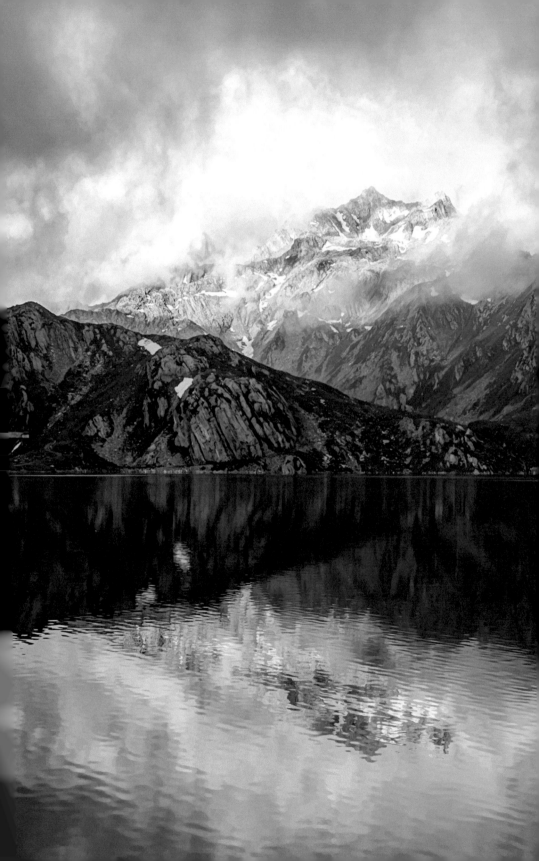

Jesus Loves Me

Jesus loves me! This I know,

For the Bible tells me so.

Little ones to Him belong;

They are weak, but He is strong.

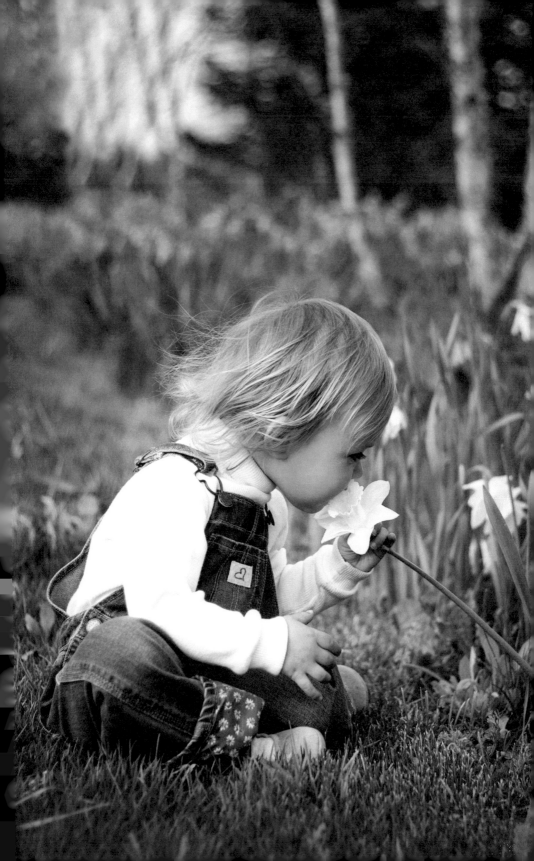

Amazing Grace

Amazing grace! How sweet the sound

That saved a wretch like me.

I once was lost, but now am found;

Was blind, but now I see.

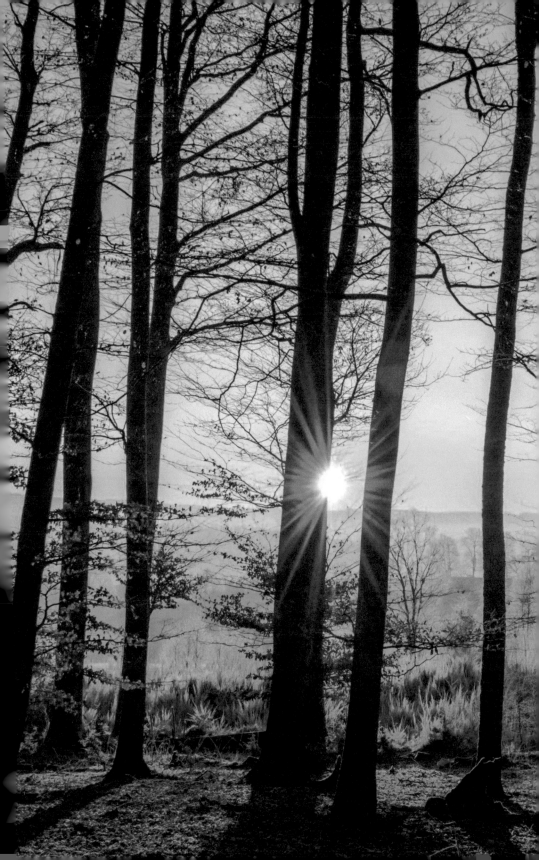

How Great Thou Art

Then sings my soul,

My Savior God, to Thee

How great Thou art!

How great Thou art!

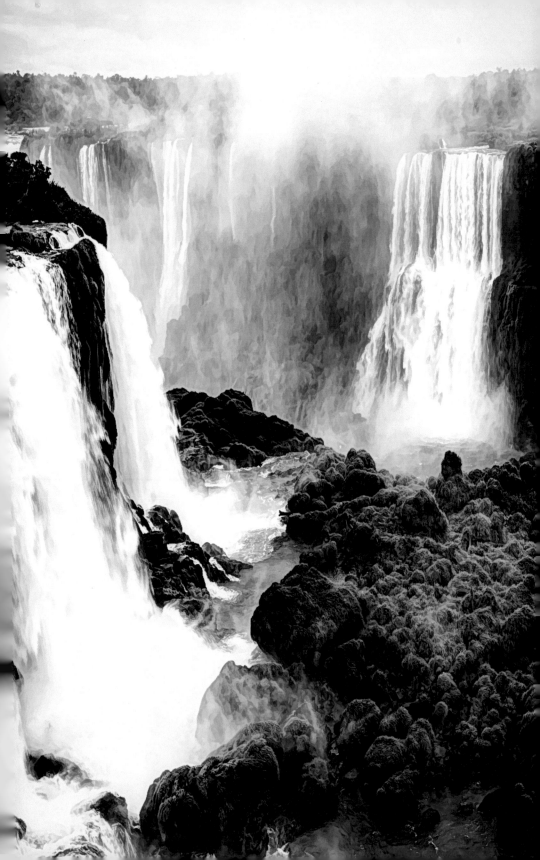

Holy, Holy, Holy

Holy, holy, holy! Lord God Almighty!

Early in the morning our song

shall rise to Thee;

Holy, holy, holy, merciful and mighty!

God in three persons, blessed Trinity!

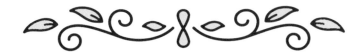

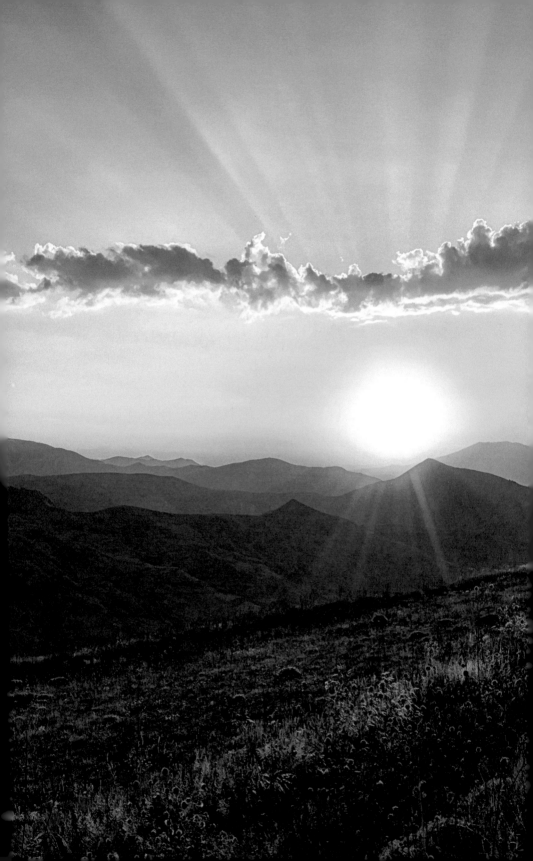

What a Friend
We Have in Jesus

What a friend we have in Jesus,

all our sins and griefs to bear!

What a privilege to carry

Everything to God in prayer!

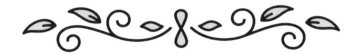

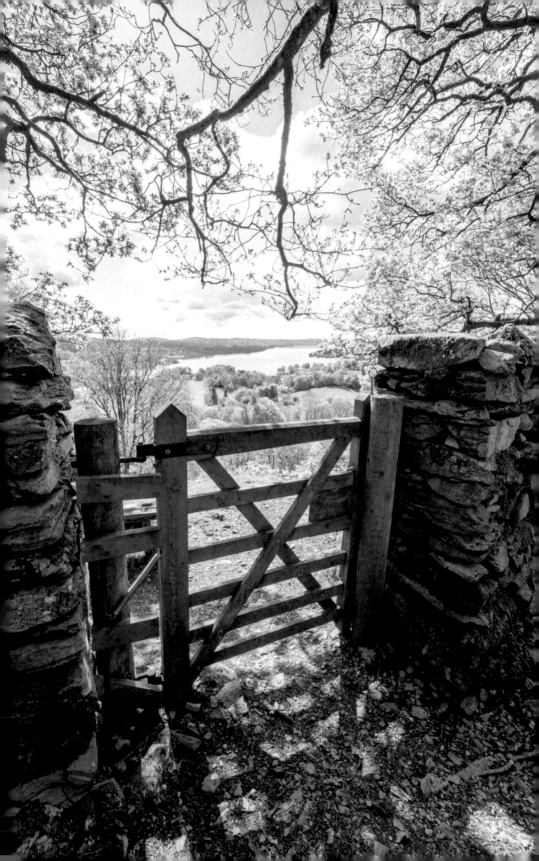

A Mighty Fortress is Our God

A mighty fortress is our God,

A bulwark never failing.

Our helper He amid the flood

Of mortal ills prevailing.

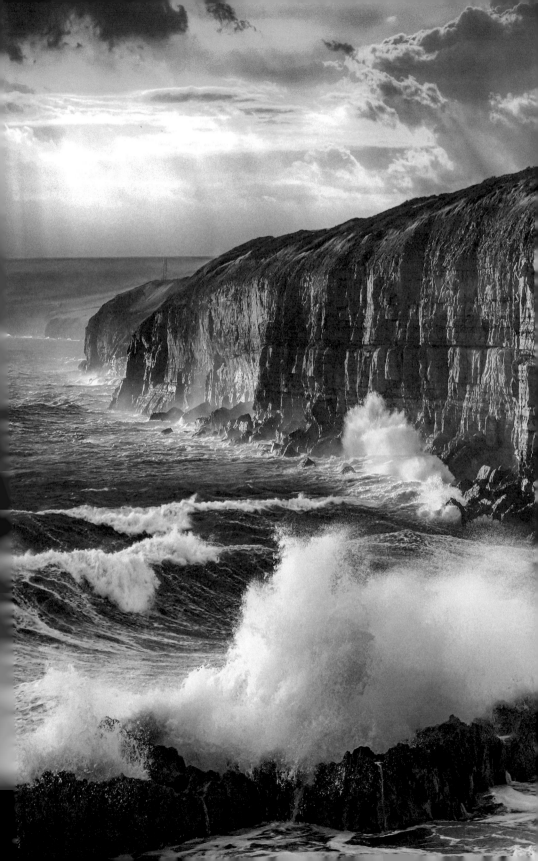

To God Be the Glory

Praise the Lord, praise the Lord,

Let the earth hear his voice!

Praise the Lord, praise the Lord,

Let the people rejoice!

O come to the Father

Through Jesus the Son,

And give him the glory,

Great things he has done!

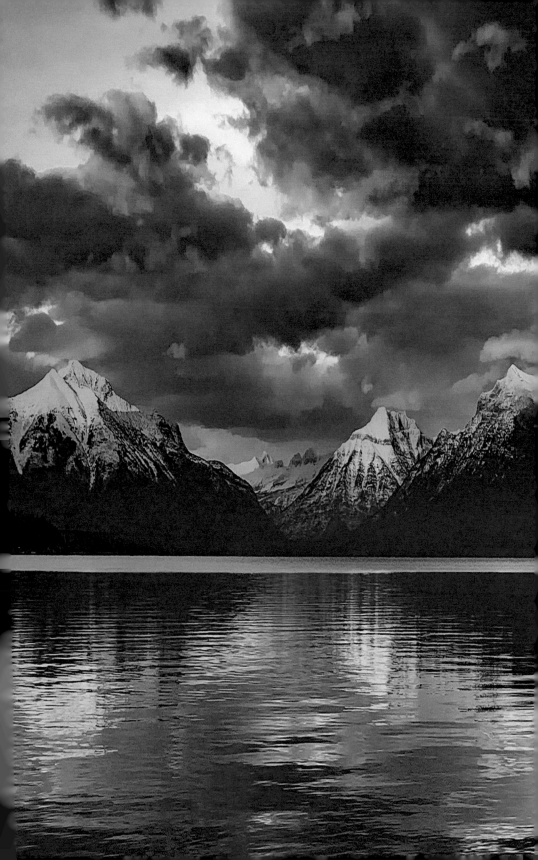

Blessed Assurance

Blessed assurance, Jesus is mine!

Oh, what a foretaste of glory divine!

Heir of salvation, purchase of God

Born of His Spirit, washed in His blood.

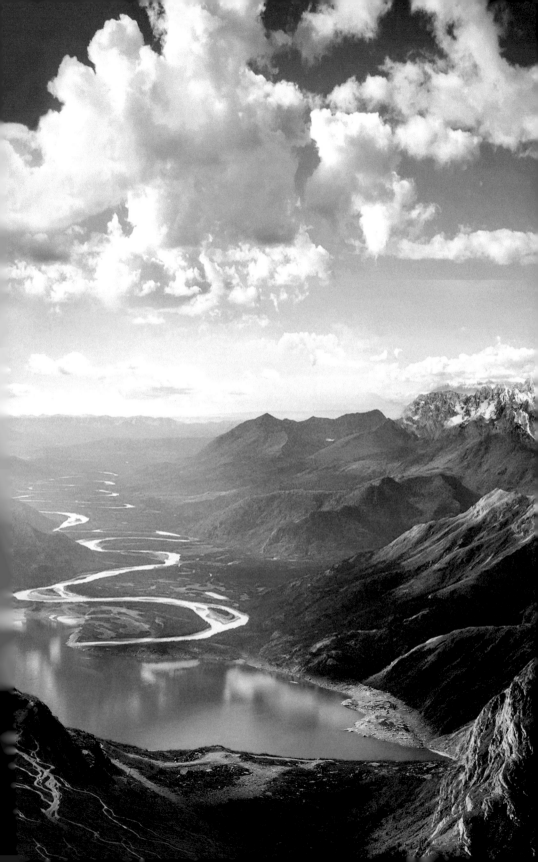

It is Well With My Soul

When peace, like a river,

Attendeth my way,

When sorrows like sea billows roll;

Whatever my lot,

Thou has taught me to say,

It is well, it is well with my soul.

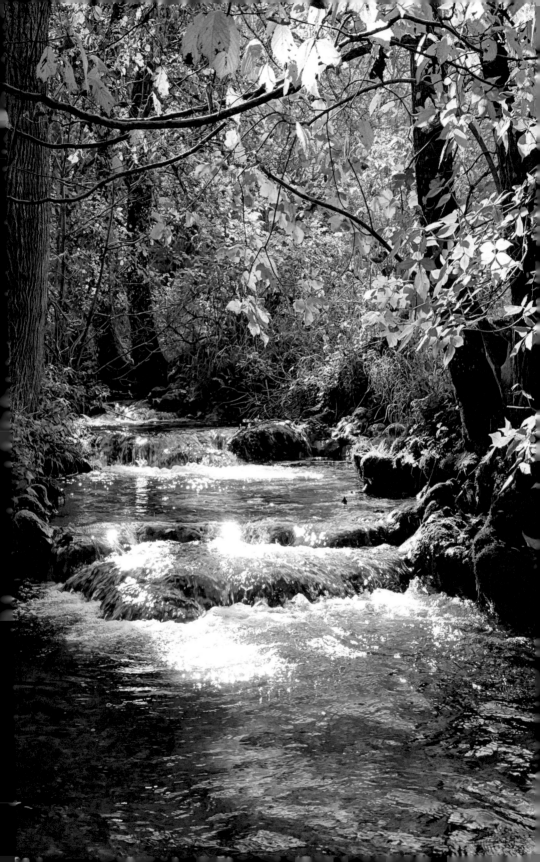

When We All Get to Heaven

When we all get to Heaven,

What a day of rejoicing that will be!

When we all see Jesus,

We'll sing and shout the victory!

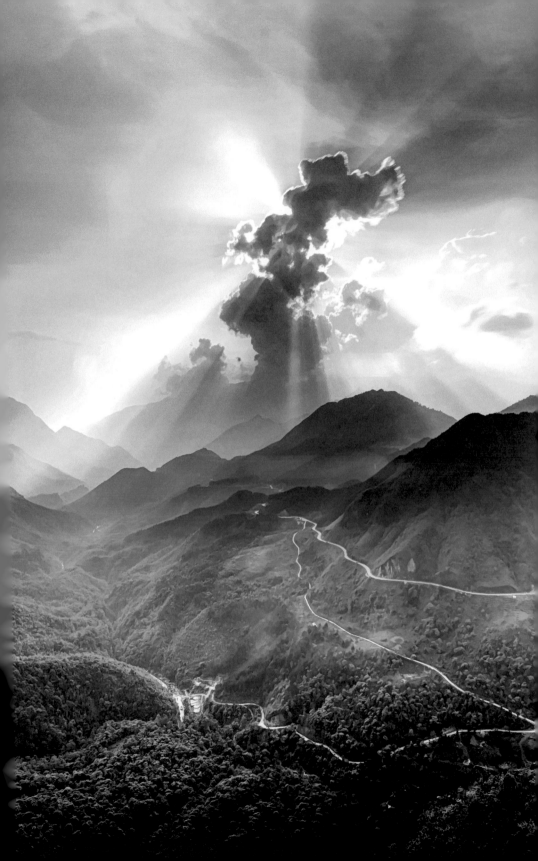

Just A Closer Walk With Thee

Just a closer walk with Thee

Grant it, Jesus, is my plea.

Daily walking close to Thee,

Let it be, dear Lord, let it be.

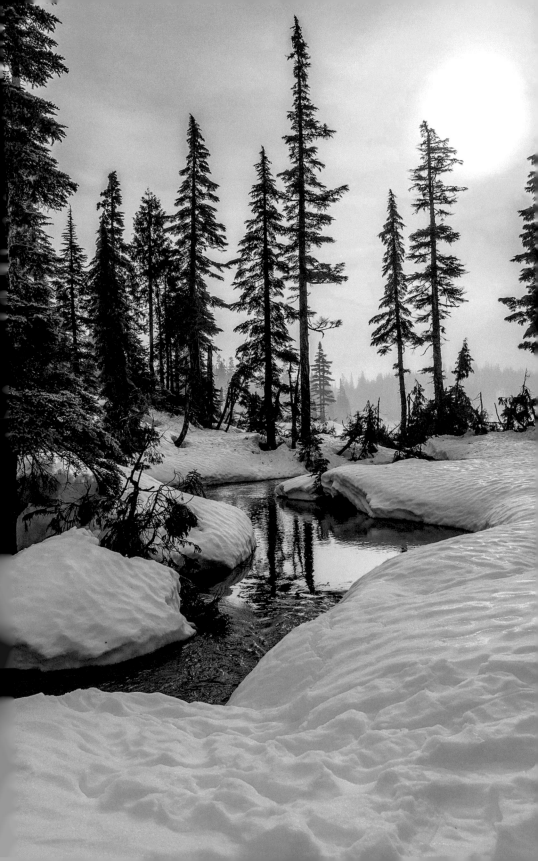

Turn Your Eyes Upon Jesus

Turn your eyes upon Jesus,

Look full in His wonderful face,

And the things of earth

Will grow strangely dim

In the light of His glory and grace.

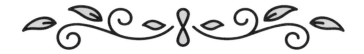

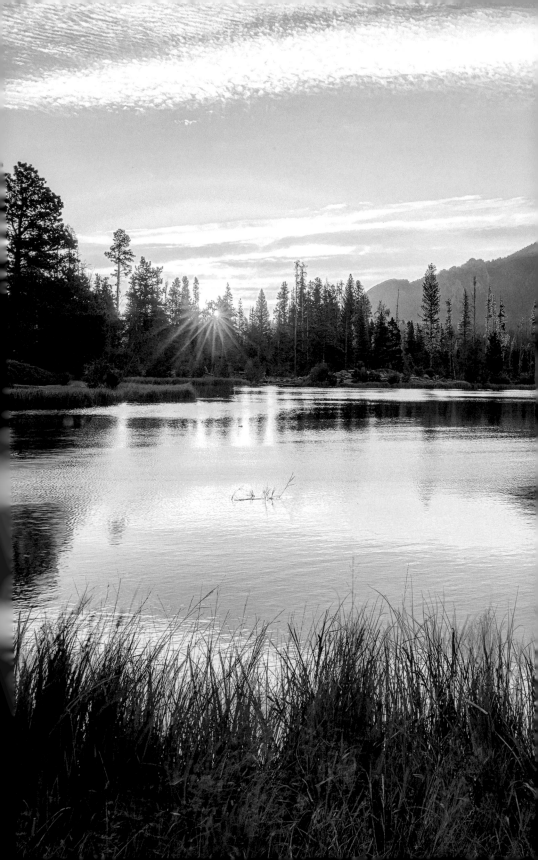

Take My Life and Let It Be

Take my life and let it be,

Consecrated, Lord, to Thee.

Take my moments and my days,

Let them flow in ceaseless praise,

Let them flow in ceaseless praise.

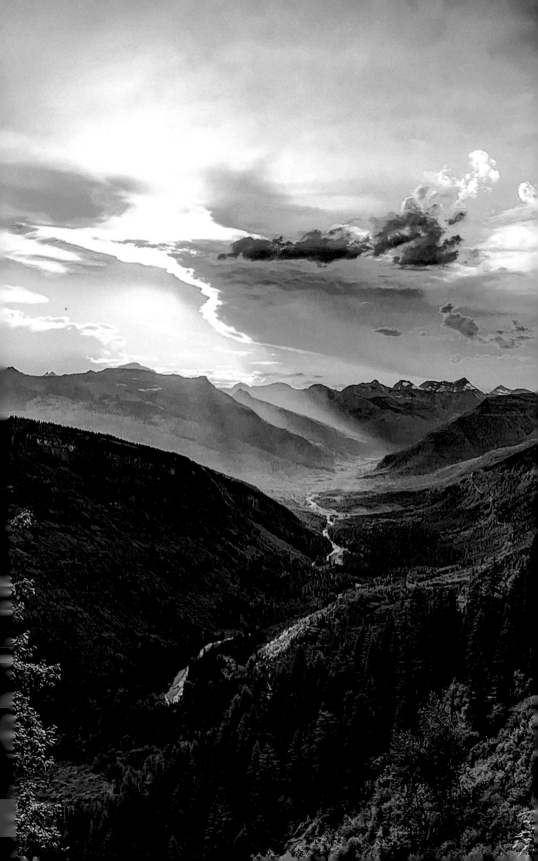

Love Lifted Me

I was sinking deep in sin,

far from the peaceful shore,

Very deeply stained within,

sinking to rise no more,

But the Master of the sea,

heard my despairing cry,

From the waters lifted me,

now safe am I.

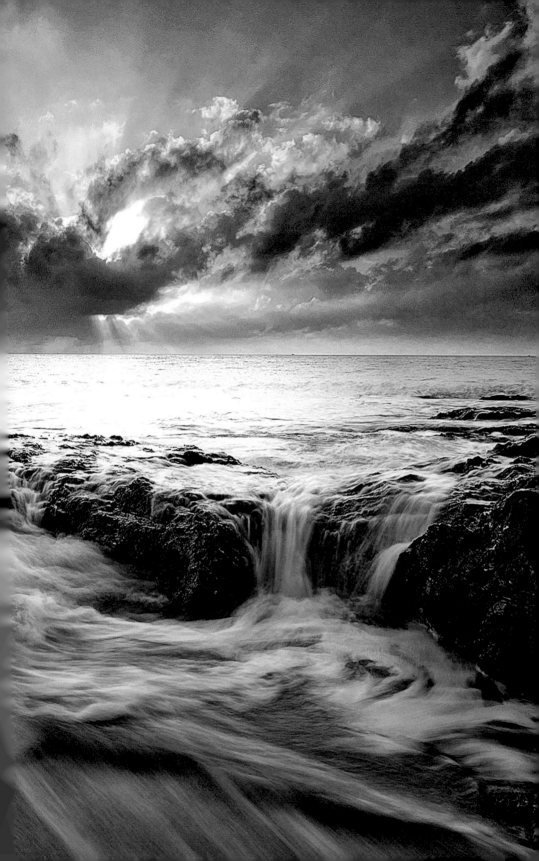

Just As I Am

Just as I am without one plea

But that thy blood was shed for me,

And that Thou bid'st me come to Thee

Oh lamb of God, I come, I come.

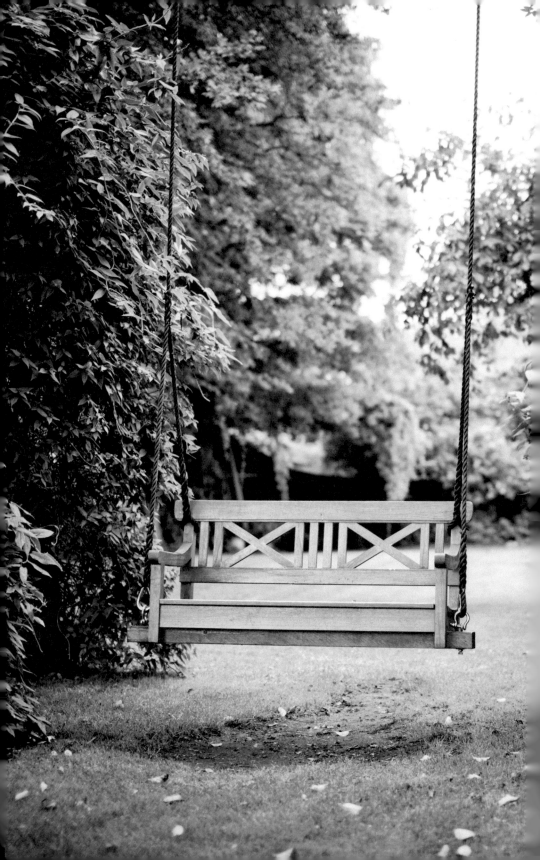

Sweet Hour of Prayer

Sweet hour of prayer!

Sweet hour of prayer!

That calls me from a world of care,

And bids me at my Father's throne

Make all my wants and wishes known.

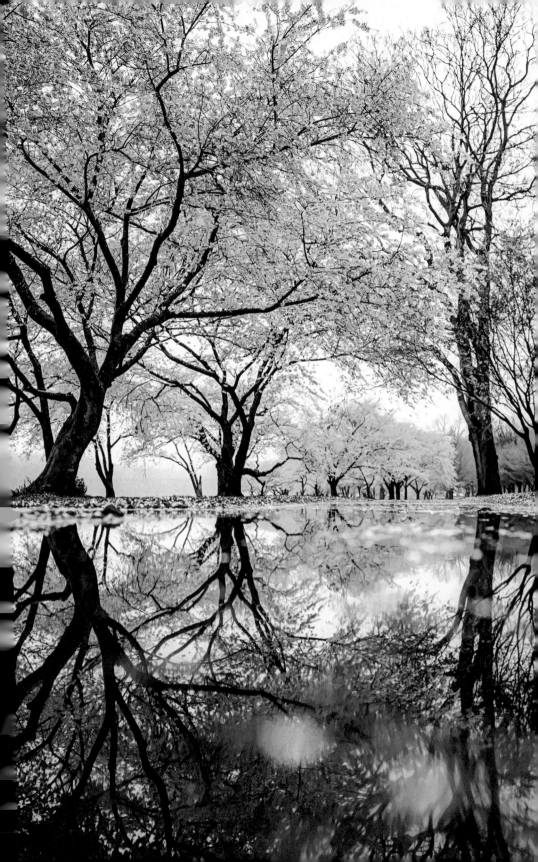

The Old Rugged Cross

On a hill far away

stood an old rugged cross

The emblem of suffering and shame;

And I love that old cross

where the dearest and best

For a world of lost sinners was slain.

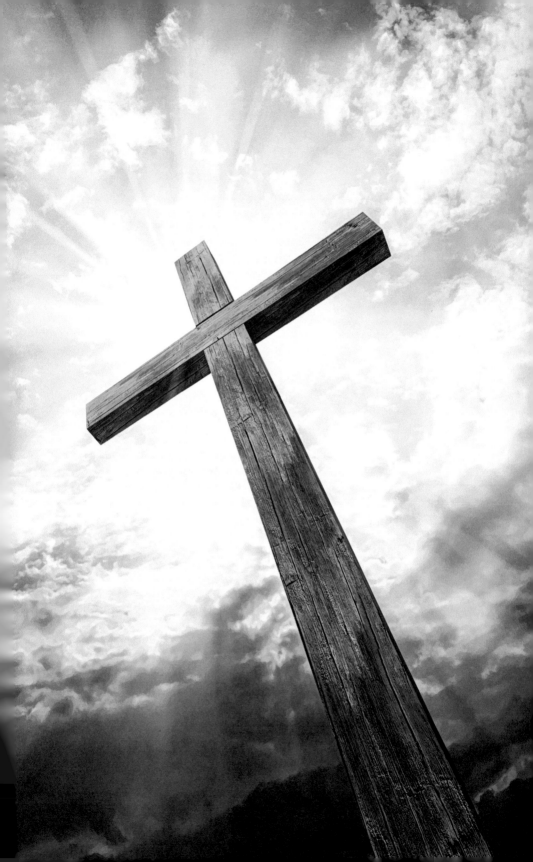

Made in the USA
Columbia, SC
27 November 2024

47483103R00024